# THE GASTRIC DIET COOKBOOK

*"Delicious and Nutritious Recipes for Improved Digestive Health"*

**Beauty Claire**

# TABLE OF CONTENTS

# INTRODUCTION TO THE GASTRIC DIET

## The Gastric System

The gastric system is a complex network of organs and tissues that are involved in the digestion of food and the absorption of nutrients to keep the body functioning. It includes the stomach, small intestine, large intestine, esophagus, and other organs.

The gastric system is responsible for breaking down food into smaller molecules and absorbing the nutrients that are needed for the body to function properly. It is also responsible for eliminating waste products from the body.

The gastric system is an important part of the digestive process and plays a vital role in maintaining health and well-being. Understanding how the gastric system works can help individuals make better food choices and improve their overall health.

The stomach is the main organ of the gastric system and is responsible for both the breakdown of food and the absorption of nutrients. The stomach produces acid and enzymes that are necessary for the breakdown of proteins, carbohydrates, and fats.

The small intestine is responsible for the majority of the absorption of nutrients and is divided into three sections: the duodenum, jejunum, and ileum. The large intestine is responsible for the absorption of water, vitamins, and minerals and for the elimination of waste products. The esophagus connects the stomach to the mouth and is responsible for the movement of food from the mouth to the stomach.

The gastric system is an integral part of the human body and is vital for maintaining health and well-being. Understanding how the gastric system works can help individuals make better food choices and lead healthier lifestyles.

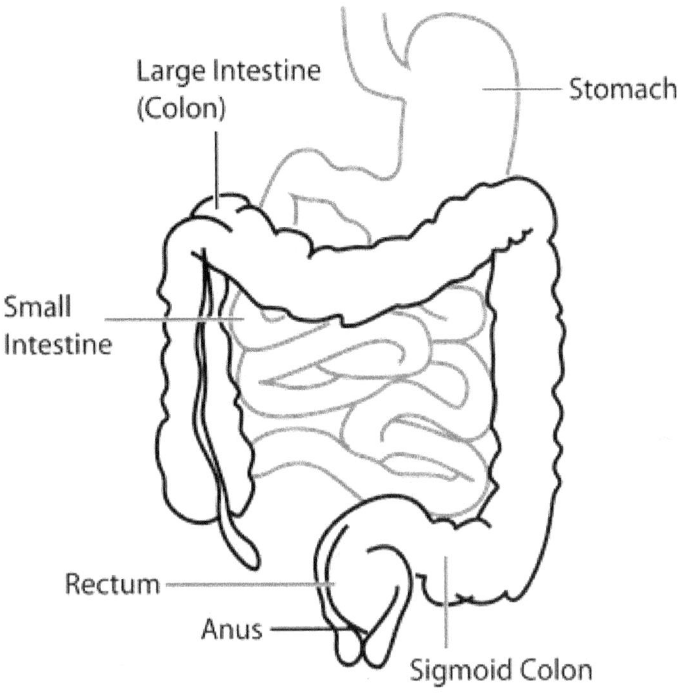



The Gastric Diet is a dietary approach created to help individuals achieve lasting weight loss and overall health. It focuses on portion control, mindful eating, and mindful lifestyle habits to create a healthy, balanced lifestyle. The diet also promotes the consumption of whole foods and encourages individuals to avoid processed and fast foods.

The diet also includes a variety of healthy fats, proteins, carbohydrates, and fiber-rich foods. The Gastric Diet is designed to help individuals reach and maintain a healthy weight, reduce cravings, and improve overall health. It is a great option for those who want to lose weight and maintain a healthy lifestyle. With the Gastric Diet, individuals can expect to lose weight without feeling deprived or hungry. This diet is also beneficial for those who suffer from digestive issues, such as gastritis, as it can help to reduce symptoms. By following the Gastric Diet, individuals can expect to see improvements in their overall health and well-being.

The Gastric Diet is an effective way to lose weight and improve health. It is a flexible approach that can be adapted to fit individual needs, goals, and preferences. It is important to note that this diet is not a one-size-fits-all approach and may not work for everyone. However, with the right guidance and support, this diet can be used to achieve lasting weight loss and improved health.

The Gastric Diet is a great option for those looking to make lasting changes to their lifestyle and improve their overall health.

# CHAPTER 1

## Problems of The Gastric System

1. Gastroesophageal reflux disease (GERD): GERD is a chronic digestive disorder that occurs when stomach acid or bile backs up into the esophagus. Symptoms of GERD include heartburn, chest pain, regurgitation, and difficulty swallowing.

2. Peptic Ulcer Disease: Peptic ulcers occur when the lining of the stomach or small intestine becomes damaged, causing an open sore. Symptoms of a peptic ulcer include abdominal pain, heartburn, nausea, vomiting, and weight loss.

3. Gastritis: Gastritis is an inflammation of the stomach lining that can cause abdominal pain, nausea, vomiting, and loss of appetite. It can be caused by bacteria, certain medications, or the long-term use of non-steroidal anti-inflammatory drugs (NSAIDs).

4. Gastroparesis: Gastroparesis is a condition in which the stomach empties too slowly, resulting in nausea, bloating, and abdominal pain. It can be caused by diabetes, certain medications, or an autoimmune disorder.

5. Irritable Bowel Syndrome (IBS): IBS is a chronic disorder of the digestive system that causes abdominal pain, bloating, gas, and changes in bowel habits. It is not known what causes IBS, although stress can be a trigger.

6. Celiac Disease: Celiac disease is an autoimmune disorder in which the ingestion of gluten damages the lining of the small intestine. Symptoms of celiac disease include diarrhea, abdominal pain, gas, and bloating.

7. Helicobacter pylori Infection: H. pylori is a type of bacteria that can live in the stomach and cause inflammation. Symptoms of an H. pylori infection include abdominal pain, nausea, vomiting, and loss of appetite.

write how dietary and lifestyle changes can help the gastric system

Dietary and lifestyle changes can help improve the health of the gastric system by:

1. Eating a balanced and nutritious diet: Eating a balanced, nutritious diet that includes plenty of fruits and vegetables, healthy proteins, and whole grains can help improve the health of the gastric system. Eating small and frequent meals

throughout the day can help prevent overeating and reduce the risk of acid reflux.

2. Avoiding certain foods: Foods that are high in fat, sugar, and processed foods can be hard for the body to digest and can cause indigestion and other gastrointestinal issues. Avoiding these foods can help improve the health of the gastric system.

3. Limiting alcohol consumption: Drinking too much alcohol can irritate the stomach lining and lead to an increased risk of developing gastritis, ulcers, and other digestive issues. Limiting alcohol consumption can help improve the health of the gastric system.

4. Regular exercise: Regular exercise can help improve the digestive system and reduce stress, which can help improve the health of the gastric system.

5. Managing stress: Stress can cause the body to produce more stomach acid, which can lead to indigestion and other gastrointestinal issues. Managing stress through activities such as yoga, meditation, and deep breathing can help improve the health of the gastric system.

# Understanding Gastric Diet.

A gastric diet is a type of diet specifically designed to help people with gastric problems, such as ulcers, acid reflux, and other digestive issues. The diet is based on the idea that avoiding certain foods can help alleviate symptoms and reduce the risk of further problems.

This type of diet usually involves avoiding irritating or hard-to-digest foods, such as those high in fat, spicy foods, caffeine, and alcohol. It also emphasizes eating smaller meals more frequently, as large meals can put extra strain on the digestive system.

Additionally, drinking plenty of fluids can help to keep the digestive system running smoothly.

Also knowing your digestive system and how it responds to different foods is important when following a gastric diet.

Knowing this will save from a lot of pain and discomfort. It is also recommended that you speak to a doctor or nutritionist before starting a gastric diet to ensure that you are doing the right thing for your specific needs.

When understanding your system and the type of food you eat, it is important to try and eat a balanced diet with a variety of foods. It is also important to try to keep your daily calorie intake within a healthy range. This can help to ensure that your digestive system is getting the nutrients it needs to stay healthy and functioning properly.

At the end of it all understanding a gastric diet is important to maintain a healthy digestive system and to prevent any further digestive issues.

The main goal of a gastric diet is to reduce the amount of strain on the digestive system and allow it to heal. This diet can help people who have a variety of digestive issues, including ulcers, irritable bowel syndrome (IBS), and Crohn's disease.

A gastric diet typically includes foods that are low in fat, high in fiber, and easy to digest. Fruits, vegetables, and lean proteins are often recommended as part of this diet. Whole grains, such as oats, barley, and brown rice, can also be helpful. Low-fat dairy products, such as plain yogurt, can also be included.

It is important to avoid certain trigger foods that can cause digestive problems. These include spicy foods, caffeine, alcohol, and certain types of fatty and sugary foods. It is also important to avoid overeating.

It is important to talk to a doctor or dietitian before starting a gastric diet. They can help create a personalized plan that is tailored to the individual's needs. They can also provide advice on how to properly follow the diet and make sure that all nutritional needs are met.

# CHAPTER 2

## What Is the Gastric Diet?

The Gastric Diet is a restrictive diet that is most commonly associated with gastric bypass surgery. It is designed to help people with obesity and other health issues to lose weight by limiting caloric intake and avoiding unhealthy foods.

This diet limits the amount of food eaten each day, with an emphasis on high-fiber, low-fat, and nutrient-dense foods.

Additionally, it encourages physical activity to help with weight loss and improve overall health.

This diet typically involves eating small meals throughout the day, avoiding unhealthy food, and focusing on nutrient-dense foods such as lean proteins, fruits, vegetables, whole grains, and low-fat dairy.

Additionally, it encourages drinking plenty of water and avoiding sugary beverages, as well as limiting alcohol intake.

The goal of the Gastric Diet is to help individuals lose weight and reduce their risk of developing serious health conditions, such as heart disease and diabetes.

By following the Gastric Diet, individuals can expect to experience weight loss, improved overall health, and improved physical and mental wellbeing.

## Benefits of The Gastric Diet

1. Improved Digestion: The gastric diet helps to improve digestion and reduce symptoms of digestive disorders such as irritable bowel syndrome.

2. Weight Loss: By limiting high-calorie and sugary foods, the gastric diet can help you lose weight.

3. Reduced Risk of Diabetes: Studies have shown that the gastric diet can help reduce the risk of developing type 2 diabetes.

4. Improved Blood Pressure: Following a gastric diet can help reduce your risk of high blood pressure.

5. Improved Cholesterol Levels: The gastric diet can help reduce cholesterol levels.

6. Reduced Risk of Heart Disease: Studies have found that the gastric diet may help to reduce the risk of heart disease.

7. Increased Energy: The gastric diet can help boost energy levels, making it easier to exercise and engage in physical activities.

8. Improved Mental Health: The gastric diet can help improve mental health by reducing stress and anxiety.

9. Improved Quality of Life: Following a gastric diet can help you lead a healthier lifestyle and improve your overall quality of life.

10. Reduced Risk of Cancer: Studies have shown that the gastric diet may help to reduce the risk of certain types of cancer.

# CHAPTER 3

## Recipes and Meal Plans

## Baked Eggplant with Tomato Sauce

**Ingredients**:

-2 medium eggplants

-2 tablespoons olive oil

-2 cloves garlic, minced

-1 can diced tomatoes

-1 teaspoon dried oregano

-1 teaspoon dried basil

-Salt and pepper to taste

-1/4 cup grated Parmesan cheese

**Instructions:**

1. Preheat the oven to 400°F.

2. Slice the eggplants into 1/4inch thick slices. Place the slices in a single layer on a baking sheet.

3. Drizzle the eggplant slices with the olive oil and sprinkle with salt and pepper.

4. Bake for 10 minutes, flipping the slices halfway through.

5. Meanwhile, heat a saucepan over medium heat. Add the garlic and cook for 1 minute.

6. Add the diced tomatoes, oregano, and basil. Simmer for 10 minutes, stirring occasionally.

7. Spread the tomato sauce over the eggplant slices. Sprinkle with the Parmesan cheese.

8. Bake for an additional 10 minutes.

9. Serve warm.

## Turkey and Zucchini Meatballs

**Ingredients:**

-1 lb. ground turkey

-1/2 cup shredded zucchini

-1/4 cup bread crumbs

-1 egg

-1/2 teaspoon garlic powder

-1 teaspoon dried oregano

-1/2 teaspoon salt

-1/4 teaspoon black pepper

**Instructions:**

1. Preheat oven to 400°F.

2. In a large bowl, combine all ingredients and mix until well combined.

3. Form the mixture into small meatballs (about 1 inch in diameter).

4. Place the meatballs on a baking sheet lined with parchment paper.

5. Bake for 20 minutes, flipping the meatballs halfway through.

6. Serve warm.

# Roasted Cauliflower and Chickpeas

**Ingredients:**

-1 head of cauliflower, cut into florets

-1 can chickpeas, drained and rinsed

-1 tablespoon olive oil

-1 teaspoon ground cumin

-1 teaspoon garlic powder

-1/2 teaspoon smoked paprika

-Salt and pepper to taste

**Instructions:**

1. Preheat oven to 425°F.

2. Place the cauliflower and chickpeas in a large bowl.

3. Drizzle the olive oil over the vegetables and sprinkle with the cumin, garlic powder, smoked paprika, salt, and pepper.

4. Toss to combine.

5. Spread the vegetables out on a baking sheet lined with parchment paper.

6. Bake for 20 minutes, stirring halfway through.

7. Serve warm.

## Mediterranean Stuffed Peppers

**Ingredients:**

-4 bell peppers, halved and seeded

-1 tablespoon olive oil

-1/2 cup diced red onion

-2 cloves garlic, minced

-1/2 cup cooked quinoa

-1/2 cup cooked brown rice

-1/2 cup crumbled feta cheese

-1/4 cup chopped fresh parsley

-1/4 cup chopped fresh mint

-1/4 cup sliced black olives

-1/4 teaspoon salt

-1/4 teaspoon black pepper

**Instructions:**

1. Preheat oven to 375°F.

2. Heat a large skillet over medium heat. Add the olive oil, red onion, and garlic. Cook until the onion is softened, about 5 minutes.

3. Remove from heat and stir in the quinoa, brown rice, feta cheese, parsley, mint, olives, salt, and pepper.

4. Stuff the peppers with the quinoa mixture. Place the peppers in a baking dish.

5. Bake for 20 minutes.

6. Serve warm.

## Zucchini and Tomato Soup

**Ingredients:**

-2 tablespoons olive oil

-1 onion, diced

-2 cloves garlic, minced

-1 teaspoon dried oregano

-4 cups vegetable broth

-2 large zucchinis, diced

-2 large tomatoes, diced

-Salt and pepper to taste

**Instructions:**

1. Heat the olive oil in a large pot over medium heat.

2. Add the onion and garlic and cook until softened, about 5 minutes.

3. Stir in the oregano, vegetable broth, zucchinis, and tomatoes.

4. Bring the mixture to a boil, then reduce heat to low and simmer for 20 minutes.

5. Carefully transfer the soup to a blender and blend until smooth.

6. Return the soup to the pot and season with salt and pepper to taste.

7. Serve warm.

## Baked Salmon with Pesto

**Ingredients:**

-4 salmon fillets

-1/4 cup pesto

-1/4 cup grated Parmesan cheese

-1/4 teaspoon garlic powder

-Salt and pepper to taste

**Instructions:**

1. Preheat oven to 400°F.

2. Line a baking sheet with parchment paper.

3. Place the salmon fillets on the baking sheet.

4. Spread the pesto over the top of each fillet.

5. Sprinkle with the Parmesan cheese, garlic powder, salt, and pepper.

6. Bake for 20 minutes, or until the salmon is cooked through.

7. Serve warm.

## Grilled Eggplant with Tahini Sauce

**Ingredients:**

-2 large eggplants, sliced into 1/2-inch rounds

-2 tablespoons olive oil

-1/4 cup tahini

-2 tablespoons lemon juice

-1 garlic clove, minced

-Salt and pepper to taste

**Instructions:**

1. Preheat the grill to medium-high heat.

2. Brush the eggplant slices with the olive oil and season with salt and pepper.

3. Grill the eggplant for 3-4 minutes per side, or until softened and lightly charred.

4. Meanwhile, in a small bowl, whisk together the tahini, lemon juice, garlic, salt, and pepper.

5. Serve the grilled eggplant with the tahini sauce.

## Baked Sweet Potato Fries

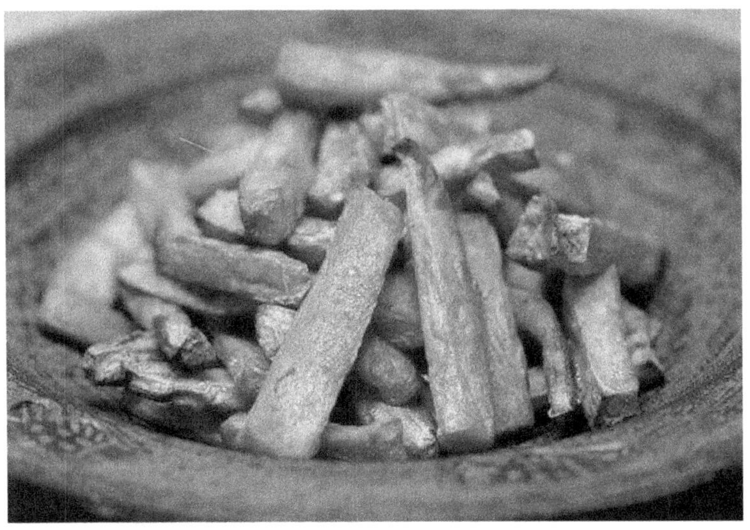

**Ingredients:**

-3 large sweet potatoes, cut into matchsticks

-2 tablespoons olive oil

-1 teaspoon dried oregano

-1/2 teaspoon garlic powder

-Salt and pepper to taste

**Instructions:**

1. Preheat oven to 425°F.

2. Line a baking sheet with parchment paper.

3. Place the sweet potato matchsticks on the baking sheet.

4. Drizzle the olive oil over the potatoes and sprinkle with the oregano, garlic powder, salt, and pepper.

5. Toss to combine.

6. Spread the potatoes out in an even layer.

7. Bake for 15 minutes, flipping the fries halfway through.

8. Serve warm.

## Baked Apples with Cinnamon

**Ingredients:**

-4 apples, cored and sliced

-2 tablespoons melted butter

-1/4 cup packed light brown sugar

-1 teaspoon ground cinnamon

-1/4 teaspoon ground nutmeg

**Instructions:**

1. Preheat oven to 375°F.

2. Place the apples in a baking dish.

3. Drizzle the melted butter over the apples.

4. In a small bowl, combine the brown sugar, cinnamon, and nutmeg. Sprinkle the mixture over the apples.

5. Bake for 20 minutes, stirring halfway through.

6. Serve warm.

## Cauliflower Rice Pilaf

**Ingredients:**

-1 head of cauliflower, cut into florets

-2 tablespoons olive oil

-1/2 cup diced onion

-1 teaspoon dried oregano

-1/4 cup chopped fresh parsley

-1/4 cup sliced almonds

-Salt and pepper to taste

**Instructions:**

1. Place the cauliflower florets in a food processor and pulse until the mixture resembles the texture of rice.

2. Heat the olive oil in a large skillet over medium heat.

3. Add the onion and cook until softened, about 5 minutes.

4. Add the cauliflower rice, oregano, and parsley. Cook, stirring occasionally, until the cauliflower is tender, about 8 minutes.

5. Stir in the almonds and season with salt and pepper to taste.

6. Serve warm.

## Baked Tofu with Vegetables

**Ingredients:**

-1 package extra-firm tofu, drained and cubed

-2 tablespoons olive oil

-1 red bell pepper, diced

-1 green bell pepper, diced

-1/2 cup sliced mushrooms

-2 cloves garlic, minced

-1 teaspoon dried oregano

-Salt and pepper to taste

**Instructions:**

1. Preheat oven to 400°F.

2. Place the tofu cubes on a baking sheet lined with parchment paper.

3. Drizzle the olive oil over the tofu and sprinkle with salt and pepper.

4. Bake for 15 minutes, flipping the cubes halfway through.

5. Meanwhile, heat a large skillet over medium heat. Add the bell peppers, mushrooms, garlic, and oregano. Cook until the vegetables are softened, about 5 minutes.

6. Add the cooked tofu to the skillet and stir to combine.

7. Serve warm.

## Baked Chicken Breasts with Spinach and Feta

**Ingredients:**

-4 boneless, skinless chicken breasts

-2 tablespoons olive oil

-2 cloves garlic, minced

-2 cups baby spinach

-1/4 cup crumbled feta cheese

-1/4 teaspoon dried oregano

-Salt and pepper to taste

**Instructions:**

1. Preheat oven to 375°F.

2. Place the chicken breasts in a baking dish.

3. Drizzle the olive oil over the chicken and sprinkle with salt and pepper.

4. Bake for 20 minutes, or until the chicken is cooked through.

5. Meanwhile, heat a large skillet over medium heat. Add the garlic and cook for 1 minute.

6. Add the spinach and cook until wilted, about 3 minutes.

7. Stir in the feta cheese and oregano and season with salt and pepper to taste.

8. Serve the chicken topped with the spinach and feta mixture.

## Greek Quinoa Salad

**Ingredients:**

-1 cup cooked quinoa

-1/2 cup diced cucumber

-1/2 cup diced tomato

-1/4 cup crumbled feta cheese

-1/4 cup sliced black olives

-2 tablespoons olive oil

-1 tablespoon lemon juice

-1 teaspoon dried oregano

-Salt and pepper to taste

**Instructions:**

1. In a large bowl, combine the quinoa, cucumber, tomato, feta cheese, and olives.

2. In a small bowl, whisk together the olive oil, lemon juice, oregano, salt, and pepper.

3. Pour the dressing over the quinoa mixture and toss to combine.

4. Serve cold or at room temperature.

## Slow Cooker Chili

**Ingredients:**

-1 tablespoon olive oil

-1 onion, diced

-2 cloves garlic, minced

-1 can diced tomatoes

-1 can black beans, drained and rinsed

-1 can kidney beans, drained and rinsed

-1 tablespoon chili powder

-1 teaspoon ground cumin

-1/2 teaspoon dried oregano

-Salt and pepper to taste

**Instructions:**

1. Heat the olive oil in a large skillet over medium heat.

2. Add the onion and garlic and cook until softened, about 5 minutes.

3. Transfer the mixture to a slow cooker.

4. Add the diced tomatoes, black beans, kidney beans, chili powder, cumin, oregano, salt, and pepper.

5. Cook on low for 4-5 hours.

6. Serve warm.

## Broiled Tilapia with Lemon

**Ingredients:**

-4 tilapia fillets

-2 tablespoons olive oil

-2 tablespoons lemon juice

-2 cloves garlic, minced

-1 teaspoon dried oregano

-Salt and pepper to taste

**Instructions:**

1. Preheat the broiler.

2. Place the tilapia fillets in a baking dish.

3. Drizzle the olive oil, lemon juice, and garlic over the fillets. Sprinkle with the oregano, salt, and pepper.

4. Broil the fish for 8-10 minutes, or until cooked through.

5. Serve warm.

## .Zucchini Noodles with Pesto

**Ingredients:**

-2 large zucchinis, spiralizer

-2 tablespoons olive oil

-1/4 cup pesto

-1/4 cup grated Parmesan cheese

-1/4 teaspoon garlic powder

-Salt and pepper to taste

**Instructions:**

1. Heat the olive oil in a large skillet over medium heat.

2. Add the zucchini noodles and cook until softened, about 5 minutes.

3. Stir in the pesto, Parmesan cheese, garlic powder, salt, and pepper.

4. Serve warm.

## Baked Falafel

**Ingredients:**

-1 can chickpeas, drained and rinsed

-1/2 cup chopped onion

-2 cloves garlic, minced

-2 tablespoons olive oil

-1 tablespoon lemon juice

-1 teaspoon ground cumin

-1/2 teaspoon ground coriander

-1/4 teaspoon dried oregano

-Salt and pepper to taste

**Instructions:**

1. Preheat oven to 375°F.

2. Place the chickpeas, onion, garlic, olive oil, lemon juice, cumin, coriander, oregano, salt, and pepper in a food processor. Process until the mixture is smooth.

3. Form the mixture into small balls (about 1 inch in diameter).

4. Place the falafel on a baking sheet lined with parchment paper.

5. Bake for 20 minutes, flipping the falafel halfway through.

6. Serve warm.

## Baked Fish with Tomatoes and Herbs

**Ingredients:**

-4 white fish fillets

-2 tablespoons olive oil

-1/4 cup diced tomatoes

-1 teaspoon dried oregano

-1 teaspoon dried basil

-1/2 teaspoon garlic powder

-Salt and pepper to taste

**Instructions:**

1. Preheat oven to 375°F.

2. Place the fish fillets in a baking dish.

3. Drizzle the olive oil over the fillets and sprinkle with the tomatoes, oregano, basil, garlic powder, salt, and pepper.

4. Bake for 20 minutes, or until the fish is cooked through.

5. Serve warm.

# Roasted Vegetable Salad

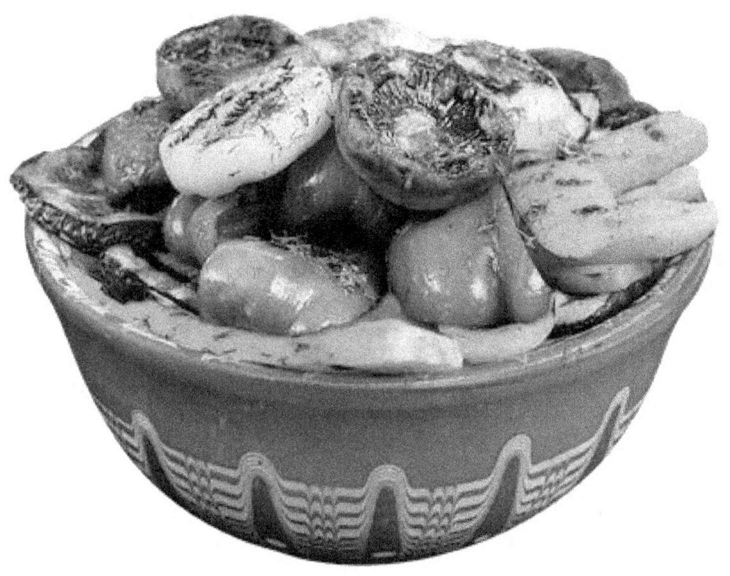

**Ingredients:**

-1 large sweet potato, diced

-1 large red bell pepper, diced

-1 large yellow bell pepper, diced

-1 large red onion, diced

-2 tablespoons olive oil

-1/4 teaspoon dried oregano

-1/4 teaspoon garlic powder

-Salt and pepper to taste

**Instructions:**

1. Preheat oven to 400°F.

2. Place the sweet potato, bell peppers, and onion in a large bowl.

3. Drizzle the olive oil over the vegetables and sprinkle with the oregano, garlic powder, salt, and pepper.

4. Toss to combine.

5. Spread the vegetables out on a baking sheet lined with parchment paper.

6. Bake for 25 minutes, stirring halfway through.

7. Serve warm or at room temperature.

## Quinoa Stuffed Peppers

**Ingredients:**

-4 bell peppers, halved and seeded

-1 tablespoon olive oil

-1/2 cup diced onion

-2 cloves garlic, minced

-1 cup cooked quinoa

-1/2 cup cooked black beans

-1/2 cup corn

-1/4 teaspoon cumin

-1/4 teaspoon chili powder

-Salt and pepper to taste

**Instructions:**

1. Preheat oven to 375°F.

2. Heat the olive oil in a large skillet over medium heat.

3. Add the onion and garlic and cook until softened, about 5 minutes.

4. Stir in the quinoa, black beans, corn, cumin, chili powder, salt, and pepper. Cook for 2-3 minutes.

5. Stuff the peppers with the quinoa mixture. Place the peppers in a baking dish.

6. Bake for 20 minutes.

7. Serve warm.

## Baked Tofu with Coconut Curry

**Ingredients:**

-1 package extra-firm tofu, drained and cubed

-1 tablespoon olive oil

-1/4 cup coconut milk

-1 tablespoon Thai red curry paste

-1 teaspoon ground ginger

-1/2 teaspoon garlic powder

-Salt and pepper to taste

**Instructions:**

1. Preheat oven to 400°F.

2. Place the tofu cubes on a baking sheet lined with parchment paper.

3. Drizzle the olive oil over the tofu and sprinkle with salt and pepper.

4. Bake for 15 minutes, flipping the cubes halfway through.

5. Meanwhile, heat a large skillet over medium heat. Add the coconut milk, red curry paste, ginger, and garlic powder. Simmer for 5 minutes.

6. Add the cooked tofu to the skillet and stir to combine.

7. Serve warm.

## Roasted Eggplant with Parsley and Feta

**Ingredients:**

-2 large eggplants, cut into 1/2-inch slices

-2 tablespoons olive oil

-1/4 cup crumbled feta cheese

-1/4 cup chopped fresh parsley

-Salt and pepper, to taste

**Instructions:**

1. Preheat oven to 375°F.

2. Line a baking sheet with foil and spread eggplant slices in a single layer.

3. Drizzle olive oil over eggplant slices and season with salt and pepper.

4. Bake in preheated oven for 25 minutes, flipping halfway through.

5. Remove eggplant from oven and sprinkle with feta cheese and parsley.

6. Bake for an additional 5 minutes, or until feta cheese is melted.

7. Serve warm.

## Cauliflower Rice with Broccoli and Mushrooms

**Ingredients:**

-1 head of cauliflower, riced

-1 cup broccoli florets

-1 cup sliced mushrooms

-2 tablespoons olive oil

-Salt and pepper, to taste

**Instructions:**

1. Heat olive oil in a large skillet over medium heat.

2. Add mushrooms and broccoli to the skillet.

3. Cook for 5 minutes, stirring occasionally.

4. Add rice cauliflower to the skillet and season with salt and pepper.

5. Cook for another 5 minutes, stirring occasionally, until vegetables are tender.

6. Serve warm.

## Poached Salmon with Cucumber Salsa

**Ingredients:**

-2 salmon fillets

-1 cup diced cucumber

-1/2 cup diced red onion

-1/4 cup diced tomatoes

-2 tablespoons chopped fresh cilantro

-1 tablespoon olive oil

-Juice of 1 lime

-Salt and pepper, to taste

**Instructions:**

1. Fill a large pot with 2 inches of water and bring to a boil over high heat.

2. Reduce heat to low, then add salmon fillets.

3. Poach salmon for 10 minutes, or until cooked through.

4. Meanwhile, combine cucumber, red onion, tomatoes, cilantro, olive oil, and lime juice in a bowl.

5. Season with salt and pepper, to taste.

6. Remove salmon from pot and flake with a fork.

7. Serve salmon with cucumber salsa.

## Greek Yogurt with Fresh Berries

**Ingredients:**

-2 cups plain Greek yogurt

-1 cup fresh blueberries

-1 cup fresh raspberries

-1/4 cup honey

**Instructions:**

1. Combine Greek yogurt, blueberries and raspberries in a bowl.

2. Drizzle honey over yogurt mixture.

3. Serve chilled.

## . Tofu Stir-Fry with Bell Peppers

**Ingredients:**

-1 block extra-firm tofu, cubed

-1 tablespoon olive oil

-1 red bell pepper, diced

-1 green bell pepper, diced

-1/4 cup diced onion

-1/4 cup diced carrots

-1 tablespoon soy sauce

-Salt and pepper, to taste

**Instructions:**

1. Heat olive oil in a large skillet over medium heat.

2. Add tofu cubes, bell peppers, onion, and carrots to the skillet.

3. Cook for 5 minutes, stirring occasionally.

4. Add soy sauce and season with salt and pepper.

5. Cook for an additional 5 minutes, or until vegetables are tender.

6. Serve warm.

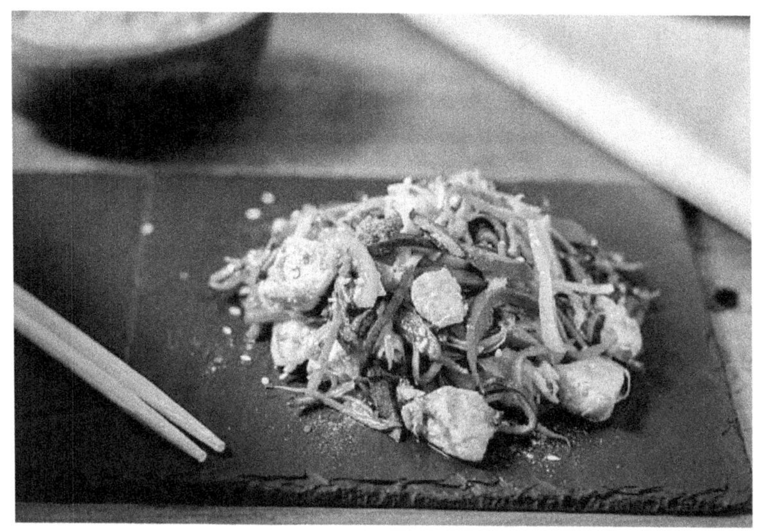

## Zucchini Noodles with Avocado Sauce

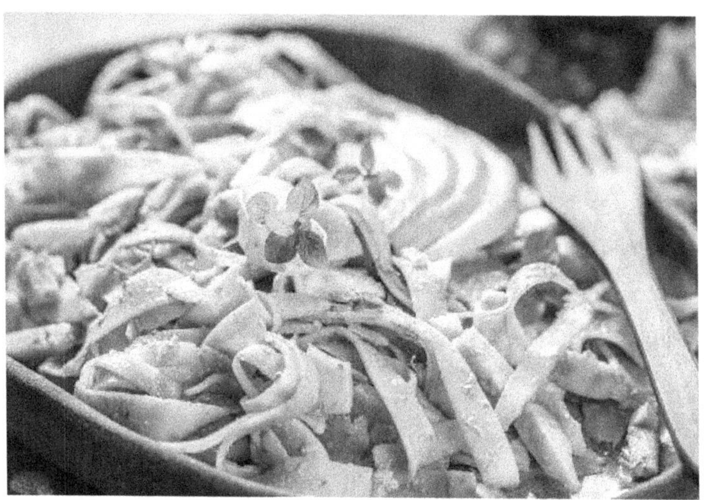

**Ingredients:**

-2 zucchinis, spiralizer

-1 avocado, pitted and peeled

-1/4 cup plain Greek yogurt

-2 tablespoons olive oil

-2 tablespoons chopped fresh cilantro

-1 teaspoon garlic powder

-Salt and pepper, to taste

**Instructions:**

1. Place spiralizer zucchini noodles in a large bowl.

2. In a blender, combine avocado, Greek yogurt, olive oil, cilantro, and garlic powder. Blend until smooth.

3. Pour avocado sauce over zucchini noodles and season with salt and pepper.

4. Toss to combine.

5. Serve chilled.

# Tomato Soup with Basil

**Ingredients**:

-2 tablespoons olive oil

-1 onion, diced

-3 cloves garlic, minced

-2 cans diced tomatoes

-2 cups vegetable broth

-1/4 cup chopped fresh basil

-Salt and pepper, to taste

**Instructions:**

1. Heat olive oil in a large pot over medium heat.

2. Add onion and garlic and cook for 5 minutes, stirring occasionally.

3. Add diced tomatoes and vegetable broth and bring to a boil.

4. Reduce heat to low and simmer for 10 minutes.

5. Add basil and season with salt and pepper.

6. Puree soup with an immersion blender until smooth.

7. Serve warm.

## Baked Apples with Cinnamon

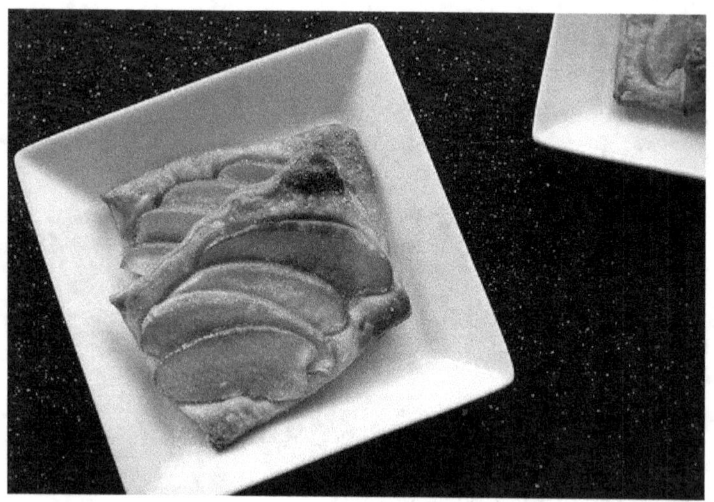

**Ingredients:**

-4 apples, cored

-1/4 cup light brown sugar

-1 teaspoon ground cinnamon

-1/4 cup water

**Instructions:**

1. Preheat oven to 375°F.

2. Place apples in a baking dish.

3. In a small bowl, mix together brown sugar and cinnamon.

4. Sprinkle brown sugar mixture over apples.

5. Pour water into the baking dish.

6. Bake for 25 minutes, or until apples are tender.

7. Serve warm.

## Lentil Stew with Kale

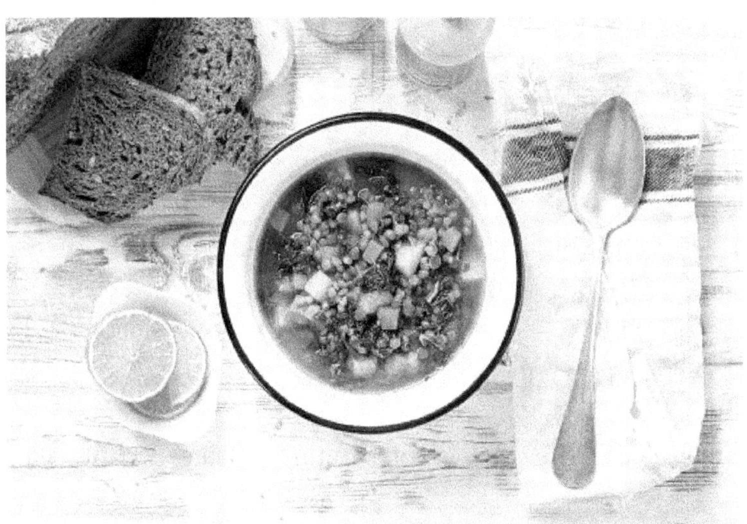

**Ingredients:**

-1 tablespoon olive oil

-1 onion, diced

-3 cloves garlic, minced

-1 cup dried lentils

-4 cups vegetable broth

-1 teaspoon ground cumin

-1/2 teaspoon smoked paprika

-1/2 teaspoon dried oregano

-3 cups chopped kale

-Salt and pepper, to taste

**Instructions:**

1. Heat olive oil in a large pot over medium heat.

2. Add onion and garlic and cook for 5 minutes, stirring occasionally.

3. Add lentils, vegetable broth, cumin, paprika, and oregano.

4. Bring to a boil, then reduce heat to low and simmer for 25 minutes, or until lentils are tender.

5. Add kale and season with salt and pepper.

6. Simmer for an additional 10 minutes, or until kale is wilted.

7. Serve warm.

# Chapter 4

## Meal Planning and Grocery Shopping

1. Start each meal with a lean protein, such as skinless chicken, fish, tofu, or eggs.

2. Incorporate plenty of vegetables, such as leafy greens, broccoli, cauliflower, and peppers.

3. Choose complex carbohydrates, like whole-grain bread, oats, or quinoa.

4. Include healthy fats, like olive oil and avocados.

5. Avoid processed and high-fat foods, such as fried foods, processed meats, and sugary treats.

Grocery Shopping:

1. Choose lean proteins, such as skinless chicken, fish, tofu, and eggs.

2. Buy plenty of fresh vegetables, such as leafy greens, broccoli, cauliflower, and peppers.

3. Look for whole-grain bread, oats, quinoa, and other complex carbohydrates.

4. Select healthy fats, like olive oil and avocados.

5. Avoid processed and high-fat foods, like fried foods, processed meats, and sugary treats.

## Breakfast Recipes

1. Overnight oats with blueberries: Combine ½ cup oats, 1 cup almond milk, 2 tablespoons chia seeds, and 1/4 teaspoon cinnamon in a bowl. Stir in 1/4 cup blueberries, cover, and refrigerate overnight.

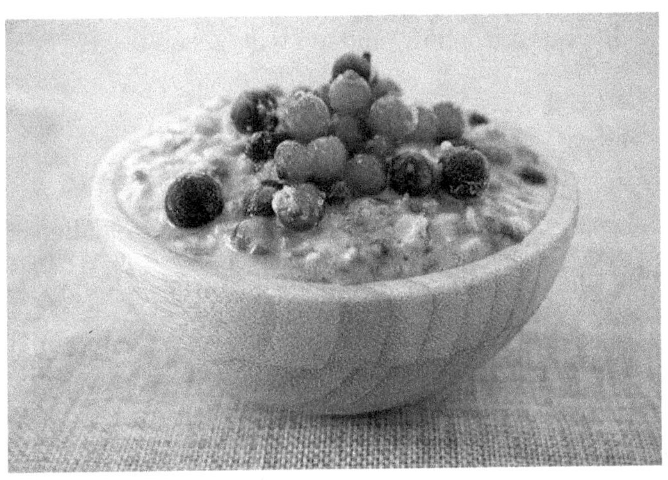

2. Avocado & Egg Toast: Toast two slices of whole-wheat bread. Top each slice with a mashed-up half of a ripe avocado and a fried egg.

3. Egg Muffins: Preheat oven to 350 degrees. Spray a muffin tin with cooking spray. Scramble 6 eggs with a dash of salt and pepper. Divide eggs among 6 muffin cups. Bake for 15 minutes.

4. Greek Yogurt Parfait: Layer ½ cup Greek yogurt, ¼ cup fresh berries, 1 tablespoon nuts and 1 tablespoon honey in a parfait glass.

5. Smoothie Bowl: Blend 1 banana, ½ cup frozen berries, ¼ cup almond milk and 1 teaspoon honey in a blender until smooth. Pour into a bowl and top with ¼ cup toasted coconut flakes.

6. Egg-White Frittata: Preheat oven to 350 degrees. Spray a 9-inch pie plate with cooking spray. Whisk together 8 egg whites and ¼ cup low-fat milk. Stir in 1 cup cooked vegetables and ½ cup low-fat cheese. Bake for 30 minutes.

7. Turkey Sausage & Veggie Scramble: Heat 1 teaspoon olive oil in a skillet over medium-high heat. Add ½ cup chopped turkey sausage and 1 cup chopped vegetables. Cook for 5 minutes, stirring occasionally. Whisk together 4 egg whites and ¼ cup low-fat milk; pour over the sausage and veggies. Cook until the egg whites are set, about 5 minutes.

8. Zucchini & Cheese Frittata: Preheat oven to 350 degrees. Spray a 9-inch pie plate with cooking spray. Whisk together 8 egg whites and ¼ cup low-fat milk. Stir in 1 cup cooked zucchini, ½ cup low-fat cheese and 1 tablespoon fresh herbs. Bake for 30 minutes.

9. Banana Oat Pancakes: In a bowl, combine ½ cup oats, 2 tablespoons chia seeds, ½ cup mashed banana, 1 egg white, and 2 tablespoons almond milk. Heat a greased skillet over medium heat and cook pancakes for a few minutes on each side.

10. Sweet Potato Hash: Heat 1 teaspoon olive oil in a skillet over medium-high heat. Add 1 cup diced sweet potatoes and 1 cup diced vegetables. Cook for 8-10 minutes, stirring occasionally. Add 2 scrambled egg whites and cook until the egg whites are set.

11. Healthy Oatmeal Muffins: Preheat oven to 350 degrees. Spray a muffin tin with cooking spray. In a bowl, combine ½ cup oats, 2 tablespoons chia seeds, ½ cup mashed banana, 1 egg white, 1 teaspoon honey, and 2 tablespoons almond milk. Divide the batter among 6 muffin cups. Bake for 20 minutes.

12. Kale & Mushroom Omelet: Heat 1 teaspoon olive oil in a skillet over medium-high heat. Add 1 cup chopped kale and 1 cup chopped mushrooms. Cook for 5 minutes, stirring occasionally.

Whisk together 4 egg whites and ¼ cup low-fat milk; pour over the kale and mushrooms. Cook until the egg whites are set, about 5 minutes.

13. Spinach & Cheese Egg Bake: Preheat oven to 350 degrees. Spray a 9-inch pie plate with cooking spray. Whisk together 8 egg whites and ¼ cup low-fat milk. Stir in 1 cup cooked spinach, ½ cup low-fat cheese and 1 tablespoon fresh herbs. Bake for 30 minutes.

14. Bacon & Egg Sandwich: Toast two slices of whole-wheat bread. Top one slice with 2 slices of cooked bacon, 1 fried egg and 1 slice of cheese.

15. Steel-Cut Oats: Bring 1 cup steel-cut oats, 2 cups of water, and a dash of salt to a boil. Reduce the heat to low and simmer for 20 minutes. Stir in a teaspoon of honey, a pinch of cinnamon, and ½ cup of your favorite fruit.

16. Quinoa Bowl: Cook ½ cup quinoa according to package instructions. Top with ½ cup cooked vegetables, 1 scrambled egg white, and 1 tablespoon of your favorite dressing.

17. Turkey Bacon & Cheese Omelet: Heat 1 teaspoon olive oil in a skillet over medium-high heat. Add 2 slices cooked turkey bacon and ½ cup cooked vegetables. Cook for 5 minutes, stirring occasionally.

Whisk together 4 egg whites and ¼ cup low-fat milk; pour over the turkey bacon and vegetables. Cook until the egg whites are set, about 5 minutes. Add 1 slice of cheese and cook until melted.

18. Sweet Potato Burrito: Heat 1 teaspoon olive oil in a skillet over medium-high heat. Add ½ cup mashed sweet potatoes and 1 cup cooked vegetables. Cook for 5 minutes, stirring occasionally. Wrap up in a whole-wheat tortilla and top with 1 scrambled egg white and 2 tablespoons salsa.

19. Baked Eggs with Spinach & Tomatoes: Preheat oven to 350 degrees. Grease a 9-inch pie plate. Arrange 2 cups of fresh spinach in the bottom of the plate. Top with 1 cup of chopped tomatoes and 8 cracked eggs. Bake for 15 minutes or until the eggs are set.

20. Apple Oatmeal: Combine ½ cup oats, 1 cup almond milk, 2 tablespoons chia seeds, and 1/4 teaspoon cinnamon in a bowl. Heat a greased skillet over medium heat and cook the oatmeal for a few minutes. Stir in 1 diced apple and a teaspoon of honey.

21. Turkey Sausage & Mushroom Frittata: Preheat oven to 350 degrees. Spray a 9-inch pie plate with cooking spray. Whisk together 8 egg whites and ¼ cup low-fat milk. Stir in ½ cup cooked turkey sausage, 1 cup cooked mushrooms, and ½ cup low-fat cheese. Bake for 30 minutes.

22. Banana & Almond Butter Toast: Toast two slices of whole-wheat bread. Top each slice with 1 tablespoon almond butter and ½ a sliced banana.

23. Baked Oatmeal: Preheat oven to 350 degrees. Grease a 9-inch pie plate. In a bowl, combine 1 cup oats, ½ teaspoon baking powder, 2 tablespoons chia seeds, ½ teaspoon cinnamon, 1 cup almond milk, and 2 tablespoons honey. Pour into the pie plate and top with ½ cup of your favorite fruit. Bake for 30 minutes.

24. Breakfast Burrito: Heat 1 teaspoon olive oil in a skillet over medium-high heat. Add 1 cup cooked vegetables and ½

cup cooked turkey sausage. Cook for 5 minutes, stirring occasionally. Wrap up in a whole-wheat tortilla and top with 1 scrambled egg white and 2 tablespoons salsa.

25. Veggie Omelet: Heat 1 teaspoon olive oil in a skillet over medium-high heat. Add 1 cup cooked vegetables. Cook for 5 minutes, stirring occasionally. Whisk together 4 egg whites and ¼ cup low-fat milk; pour over the vegetables. Cook until the egg whites are set, about 5 minutes.

26. Egg & Cheese Sandwich: Toast two slices of whole-wheat bread. Top one slice with a fried egg and 1 slice of cheese.

27. Oatmeal & Fruit: Combine ½ cup oats, 1 cup almond milk, 2 tablespoons chia seeds, and 1/4 teaspoon cinnamon in a bowl. Heat a greased skillet over medium heat and cook the oatmeal for a few minutes. Stir in 1/4 cup of your favorite fruit and a teaspoon of honey.

28. Egg & Potato Hash: Heat 1 teaspoon olive oil in a skillet over medium-high heat. Add 1 cup diced cooked potatoes and 1 cup cooked vegetables. Cook for 8-10 minutes, stirring occasionally. Add 2 scrambled egg whites and cook until the egg whites are set.

29. Baked Egg Cups: Preheat oven to 350 degrees. Grease a 6-cup muffin tin. Divide cooked vegetables and turkey sausage among the muffin cups. Crack an egg into each cup. Bake for 15 minutes.

30. Yogurt Parfait: Layer ½ cup plain yogurt, ¼ cup fresh berries, 1 tablespoon nuts, half tablespoon of granola and 1 tablespoon honey in a parfait glass.

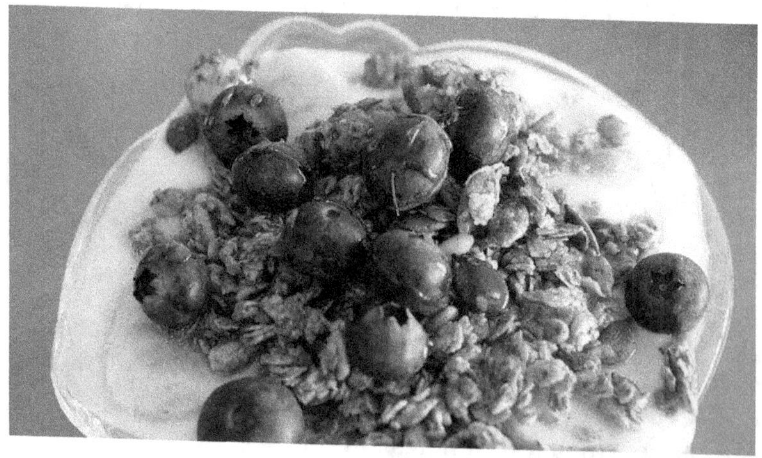

## Lunch Recipes

1. Cucumber and Tomato Salad: Slice one cucumber, two tomatoes, and two radishes. Toss with a tablespoon of olive oil, a pinch of salt, and a squeeze of fresh lemon juice. Serve chilled.

2. Baked Tilapia with Asparagus: Preheat oven to 375°F. Place one tilapia fillet and one bunch of asparagus on a baking sheet. Drizzle with olive oil and season with salt and pepper. Bake for 20 minutes.

3. Omelet with Mushrooms and Spinach: In a bowl, whisk two eggs and a tablespoon of milk. Heat a non-stick skillet over medium heat and add a tablespoon of olive oil. Add one cup of sliced mushrooms and a cup of spinach. Pour in the egg mixture and cook until eggs are set. Flip omelet and cook for another 2 minutes. Serve hot.

4. Broiled Salmon with Herbed Quinoa: Preheat oven to broil. Place one salmon fillet on a baking sheet. Drizzle with olive oil and season with salt, pepper, and herbs. Broil for 8 minutes. Meanwhile, prepare one cup of quinoa according to package instructions.

5. Baked Salmon with Roasted Broccoli: Preheat oven to 375°F. Place one salmon fillet and one head of broccoli florets on a baking sheet. Drizzle with olive oil and season with salt and pepper. Bake for 20 minutes.

6. Stuffed Bell Peppers: Preheat oven to 375°F. Slice two bell peppers in half lengthwise. Remove seeds and ribs.

Place peppers in a baking dish. In a bowl, mix one cup cooked quinoa, one cup cooked black beans, one cup corn, ½ cup shredded cheese, and ½ cup salsa. Stuff each pepper with the quinoa mixture. Bake for 25 minutes.

7. Lentil Soup: Heat a large pot over medium heat and add a tablespoon of olive oil. Add one cup of chopped onion, one cup of chopped celery, and one cup of chopped carrots. Cook until vegetables are softened. Stir in one cup of dried lentils and four cups of vegetable broth. Simmer for 25 minutes.

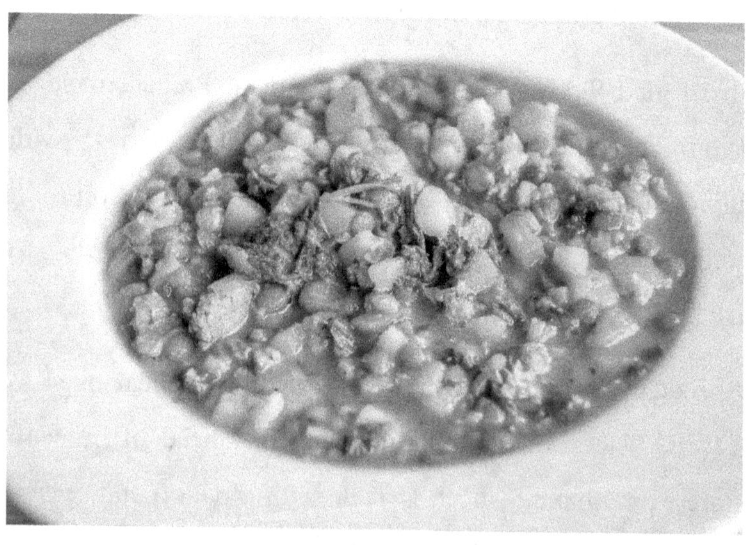

8. Quinoa Stuffed Zucchini Boats: Preheat oven to 375°F. Slice two zucchinis in half lengthwise. Remove seeds. Place zucchinis in a baking dish. In a bowl, mix one cup cooked quinoa, one cup cooked black beans, one cup corn, ½ cup shredded cheese, and ½ cup salsa. Stuff each zucchini with the quinoa mixture. Bake for 25 minutes.

9. Baked Tilapia with Roasted Tomatoes: Preheat oven to 375°F. Place one tilapia fillet and one cup of halved cherry tomatoes on a baking sheet. Drizzle with olive oil and season with salt and pepper. Bake for 20 minutes.

10. Grilled Chicken with Veggies: Preheat a grill or grill pan over medium-high heat. Place two chicken breasts on the grill. Grill for 5 minutes and then flip. Grill for another 5 minutes. Meanwhile, prepare a veggie skewer with one cup each of bell peppers and mushrooms. Grill for 5 minutes.

11. Eggplant Parmesan: Preheat oven to 375°F. Slice one eggplant into ½ inch thick slices. Place eggplant slices on a baking sheet. Drizzle with olive oil and season with salt and pepper. Bake for 20 minutes. Meanwhile, prepare tomato sauce. To assemble, layer eggplant slices in a baking dish.

Top with tomato sauce and ¼ cup of grated cheese. Bake for 10 minutes.

12. Gazpacho: In a blender, combine two cups of tomato juice, one cup of chopped cucumber, one cup of chopped bell pepper, one cup of chopped onion, one garlic clove, two tablespoons of olive oil, and one tablespoon of red wine vinegar. Blend until smooth. Serve chilled.

13. Lentil Salad: In a bowl, mix one cup cooked lentils, one cup cooked quinoa, one cup cooked corn, one cup diced tomatoes, one cup chopped cucumber, one cup chopped bell pepper, and one cup chopped onion. Toss with two tablespoons of olive oil, two tablespoons of red wine vinegar, and a pinch of salt.

14. Stuffed Eggplant: Preheat oven to 375°F. Slice one eggplant in half lengthwise. Remove seeds and ribs. Place eggplant in a baking dish. In a bowl, mix one cup cooked quinoa, one cup cooked black beans, one cup corn, ½ cup shredded cheese, and ½ cup salsa. Stuff each eggplant with the quinoa mixture. Bake for 25 minutes.

15. Baked Salmon with Roasted Asparagus: Preheat oven to 375°F. Place one salmon fillet and one bunch of asparagus

on a baking sheet. Drizzle with olive oil and season with salt and pepper. Bake for 20 minutes.

16. Grilled Chicken with Roasted Sweet Potatoes: Preheat a grill or grill pan over medium-high heat. Place two chicken breasts on the grill. Grill for 5 minutes and then flip. Grill for another 5 minutes. Meanwhile, prepare a veggie skewer with one cup of cubed sweet potatoes. Grill for 5 minutes.

17. Stuffed Acorn Squash: Preheat oven to 375°F. Cut two acorn squashes in half lengthwise. Remove seeds and ribs. Place squash in a baking dish. In a bowl, mix one cup cooked quinoa, one cup cooked black beans, one cup corn, ½ cup shredded cheese, and ½ cup salsa. Stuff each squash with the quinoa mixture. Bake for 25 minutes.

18. Quinoa Bowl: In a bowl, mix one cup cooked quinoa, one cup cooked black beans, one cup cooked corn, ½ cup diced tomatoes, one cup chopped cucumber, one cup chopped bell pepper, one cup chopped onion, two tablespoons of olive oil, two tablespoons of red wine vinegar, and a pinch of salt. Serve chilled.

19. Baked Tilapia with Roasted Broccoli: Preheat oven to 375°F. Place one tilapia fillet and one head of broccoli

florets on a baking sheet. Drizzle with olive oil and season with salt and pepper. Bake for 20 minutes.

20. Tomato Soup: Heat a large pot over medium heat and add a tablespoon of olive oil. Add one cup of chopped onion and one garlic clove and cook until softened. Stir in two cups of tomato puree and four cups of vegetable broth. Simmer for 20 minutes.

21. Greek Salad: In a bowl, mix one cup diced tomatoes, one cup chopped cucumber, one cup chopped bell pepper, one cup chopped onion, one cup crumbled feta cheese, and two tablespoons of olive oil. Toss with a squeeze of fresh lemon juice and a pinch of salt. Serve chilled.

22. Grilled Turkey Burger: Preheat a grill or grill pan over medium-high heat. Form one pound of lean ground turkey into four patties. Grill for 5 minutes and then flip. Grill for another 5 minutes. Serve on a whole-wheat bun with lettuce, tomato, and onion.

23. Baked Salmon with Roasted Cauliflower: Preheat oven to 375°F. Place one salmon fillet and one head of cauliflower florets on a baking sheet. Drizzle with olive oil and season with salt and pepper. Bake for 20 minutes.

24. Quinoa Bowl with Avocado: In a bowl, mix one cup cooked quinoa, one cup cooked black beans, one cup cooked corn, ½ cup diced tomatoes, one cup chopped cucumber, one cup chopped bell pepper, one cup chopped onion, two tablespoons of olive oil, two tablespoons of red wine vinegar, and a pinch of salt. Top with one diced avocado. Serve chilled.

25. Eggplant Parmesan: Preheat oven to 375°F. Slice one eggplant into ½ inch thick slices. Place eggplant slices on a baking sheet. Drizzle with olive oil and season with salt and pepper. Bake for 20 minutes. Meanwhile, prepare tomato sauce. To assemble, layer eggplant slices in a baking dish. Top with tomato sauce and ¼ cup of grated cheese. Bake for 10 minutes.

26. Lentil Burgers: In a food processor, combine one cup cooked lentils, one cup cooked quinoa, one cup cooked oats, one egg, one tablespoon of olive oil, one teaspoon of garlic powder, and one teaspoon of onion powder. Pulse until combined. Form into four patties. Heat a non-stick skillet over medium heat and add a tablespoon of olive oil. Cook

patties for 5 minutes on each side. Serve on a whole-wheat bun with lettuce, tomato, and onion.

27. Baked Tilapia with Roasted Tomatoes and Zucchini: Preheat oven to 375°F. Place one tilapia fillet and one cup of halved cherry tomatoes and one cup of diced zucchini on a baking sheet. Drizzle with olive oil and season with salt and pepper. Bake for 20 minutes.

28. Greek Quinoa Bowl: In a bowl, mix one cup cooked quinoa, one cup cooked black beans, one cup cooked corn, ½ cup diced tomatoes, one cup chopped cucumber, one cup chopped bell pepper, one cup chopped onion, two tablespoons of olive oil, two tablespoons of red wine vinegar, and a pinch of salt. Top with one cup crumbled feta cheese. Serve chilled.

29. Baked Salmon with Roasted Carrots: Preheat oven to 375°F. Place one salmon fillet and one cup of chopped carrots on a baking sheet. Drizzle with olive oil and season with salt and pepper. Bake for 20 minutes.

30. Lentil Stew: Heat a large pot over medium heat and add a tablespoon of olive oil. Add one cup of chopped onion, one cup of chopped celery, and one cup of chopped carrots. Cook

until vegetables are softened. Stir in one cup of dried lentils, four cups of vegetable broth, and one cup of diced tomatoes. Simmer for 25 minutes.

## Dinner Recipes

1. Baked Salmon with Asparagus: Preheat oven to 350°F. Place a piece of salmon in a baking dish. Top with a few sprigs of asparagus and 1 tablespoon of olive oil. Bake for 15 minutes, or until the salmon is cooked through. Enjoy!

2. Grilled Chicken with Zucchini: Preheat a grill to medium-high heat. Place a few pieces of chicken on the grill. Grill for 4 minutes, then flip. Grill for an additional 4 minutes, or until cooked through. Serve with grilled zucchini slices.

3. Steamed Broccoli and Carrots: Bring a pot of water to a boil. Add 1 cup of broccoli and 1 cup of carrots. Steam for 10 minutes, or until both vegetables are tender. Enjoy!

4. Roasted Red Pepper Soup: Preheat oven to 400°F. Place 4 red peppers on a baking sheet. Roast for 25 minutes, or until the peppers are soft. Place peppers in a blender with 1 cup of vegetable stock and blend until smooth. Serve with a dollop of Greek yogurt.

**77 |THE GASTRIC DIET COOKBOOK**

5. Baked Sweet Potato Fries: Preheat oven to 425°F. Cut 2 sweet potatoes into thin strips. Place them on a lightly greased baking sheet. Drizzle with 1 tablespoon of olive oil. Bake for 20 minutes, or until fries are golden brown. Enjoy!

6. Egg White Omelet with Spinach: Heat a non-stick skillet over medium-high heat. Add 1 cup of egg whites and cook for 1 minute. Add 1 cup of spinach and cook for an additional 2 minutes, or until egg whites are cooked through. Enjoy!

7. Quinoa and Vegetable Stir Fry: Heat a skillet over medium-high heat. Add 1 tablespoon of olive oil and 1 cup of quinoa. Cook for 3 minutes, stirring occasionally. Add 1 cup of mixed vegetables and cook for an additional 5 minutes, or until vegetables are tender. Enjoy!

8. Cauliflower Rice Burrito Bowls: Heat a skillet over medium-high heat. Add 1 tablespoon of olive oil and 1 cup of cauliflower rice. Cook for 5 minutes, stirring occasionally. Add 1 cup of black beans and cook for an additional 5 minutes. Serve in a bowl topped with your favorite burrito toppings.

9. Baked Tofu with Brown Rice: Preheat oven to 350°F. Place 1 block of extra firm tofu on a baking sheet. Drizzle

with 1 tablespoon of olive oil and 1 teaspoon of garlic powder. Bake for 20 minutes, or until tofu is golden brown. Serve with 1 cup of cooked brown rice. Enjoy!

10. Greek Salad: Place 1 head of romaine lettuce in a large bowl. Add 1 cup of cherry tomatoes, 1 cucumber (sliced), 1/2 cup of Kalamata olives, 1/4 cup of feta cheese, 1/4 cup of diced red onion, and 1/4 cup of diced red bell pepper. Drizzle with 1/4 cup of olive oil and 1/4 cup of red wine vinegar. Enjoy!

11. Lentil Stew: Heat a large pot over medium-high heat. Add 1 tablespoon of olive oil and 1 cup of diced onion. Cook for 3 minutes, stirring occasionally. Add 1 cup of dried lentils and 1 quart of vegetable broth. Bring to a boil, then reduce heat and simmer for 20 minutes, or until lentils are tender. Enjoy!

12. Baked Salmon Cakes: Preheat oven to 375°F. Place 1 can of salmon in a large bowl. Add 1/2 cup of bread crumbs, 1/4 cup of diced red onion, 1/4 cup of diced red bell pepper, 1 egg, and 1 tablespoon of Italian seasoning. Mix until combined. Form into patties and place on a baking sheet. Bake for 15 minutes, or until golden brown. Enjoy!

13. Zucchini Noodles with Pesto: Heat a large skillet over medium-high heat. Add 1 tablespoon of olive oil and 1 zucchini (Spiralizer). Cook for 3 minutes, stirring occasionally. Add 1/4 cup of pesto and cook for an additional 2 minutes. Serve with a sprinkle of parmesan cheese. Enjoy!

14. Broccoli and Cheese Quiche: Preheat oven to 375°F. Place 1 9-inch unbaked pie crust in a pie dish. Spread 1 cup of broccoli florets over the crust. Sprinkle 1/2 cup of shredded cheese over the top. Whisk together 3 eggs and 1/2 cup of milk in a bowl. Pour egg mixture over the top. Bake for 25 minutes, or until quiche is golden brown. Enjoy!

15. Turkey Burgers with Sweet Potato Fries: Preheat oven to 400°F. Place 4 sweet potatoes on a baking sheet. Drizzle with 1 tablespoon of olive oil. Bake for 20 minutes, or until fries are golden brown. Place 1 lb. of ground turkey in a large bowl. Add 1/2 cup of diced onion, 1/2 teaspoon of garlic powder, 1/2 teaspoon of oregano, and 1/4 teaspoon of salt. Mix until combined. Form into patties and cook on a skillet over medium-high heat for 8 minutes on each side, or until cooked through. Serve with sweet potato fries. Enjoy!

16. Grilled Vegetable Wrap: Preheat a grill to medium-high heat. Place 1 bell pepper, 1 zucchini, and 1 onion on the grill. Grill for 4 minutes, then flip. Grill for an additional 4 minutes, or until vegetables are tender. Place vegetables in a large wrap with 1/4 cup of hummus and 1/4 cup of feta cheese. Enjoy!

17. Baked Chicken Parmesan: Preheat oven to 350°F. Place 4 chicken breasts in a baking dish. Top with 1/2 cup of marinara sauce and 1/2 cup of shredded mozzarella cheese. Bake for 25 minutes, or until chicken is cooked through. Enjoy!

18. Quinoa and Black Bean Salad: Place 1 cup of cooked quinoa in a large bowl. Add 1/2 cup of cooked black beans, 1 diced red bell pepper, 1/4 cup of diced red onion, and 1/4 cup of diced cilantro. Drizzle with 1/4 cup of olive oil and 1/4 cup of lime juice. Enjoy!

19. Roasted Brussels Sprouts: Preheat oven to 400°F. Place 1 lb. of Brussels sprouts on a baking sheet. Drizzle with 1 tablespoon of olive oil and 1 teaspoon of garlic powder. Bake for 20 minutes, or until Brussels sprouts are golden brown. Enjoy!

20. Baked Cod with Spinach: Preheat oven to 375°F. Place 4 cod fillets in a baking dish. Top with 1/2 cup of spinach and 1 tablespoon of olive oil. Bake for 20 minutes, or until cod is cooked through. Enjoy!

21. Broiled Salmon with Asparagus: Preheat oven to broil. Place a piece of salmon in a baking dish. Top with a few sprigs of asparagus and 1 tablespoon of olive oil. Broil for 8 minutes, or until salmon is cooked through. Enjoy!

22. Lentil Kale Soup: Heat a large pot over medium-high heat. Add 1 tablespoon of olive oil and 1 diced onion. Cook for 3 minutes, stirring occasionally. Add 1 cup of dried lentils, 1 quart of vegetable broth, and 1 bunch of chopped kale. Bring to a boil, then reduce heat and simmer for 20 minutes, or until lentils are tender. Enjoy!

23. Grilled Vegetable Quesadillas: Preheat a grill to medium-high heat. Place 1 bell pepper, 1 zucchini, and 1 onion on the grill. Grill for 4 minutes, then flip. Grill for an additional 4 minutes, or until vegetables are tender. Place vegetables in a large wrap with 1/4 cup of shredded cheese. Grill for 3 minutes on each side, or until quesadilla is golden brown and cheese is melted. Enjoy!

24. Baked Tofu with Brown Rice: Preheat oven to 350°F. Place 1 block of extra firm tofu on a baking sheet. Drizzle with 1 tablespoon of olive oil and 1 teaspoon of garlic powder. Bake for 20 minutes, or until tofu is golden brown. Serve with 1 cup of cooked brown rice. Enjoy!

25. Roasted Butternut Squash Soup: Preheat oven to 400°F. Place 1 large butternut squash on a baking sheet. Drizzle with 1 tablespoon of olive oil and 1 teaspoon of garlic powder. Roast for 30 minutes, or until squash is soft. Place roasted squash in a blender with 1 cup of vegetable stock and blend until smooth. Enjoy!

26. Baked Eggplant Parmesan: Preheat oven to 375°F. Place 4 eggplant slices on a baking sheet. Top each slice with 1/4 cup of marinara sauce and 1/4 cup of shredded mozzarella cheese. Bake for 25 minutes, or until eggplant is cooked through. Enjoy!

27. Turkey Stuffed Peppers: Preheat oven to 350°F. Place 4 bell peppers in a baking dish. In a large bowl, mix together 1 lb. of ground turkey, 1/2 cup of cooked quinoa, 1/2 cup of diced onion, and 1/2 cup of diced bell pepper. Stuff each bell

pepper with the turkey mixture. Bake for 25 minutes, or until peppers are tender. Enjoy!

28. Fennel and Apple Salad: Place 1 fennel bulb (shredded) in a large bowl. Add 1 apple (diced), 1/4 cup of diced red onion, and 1/4 cup of chopped walnuts. Drizzle with 1/4 cup of olive oil and 1/4 cup of apple cider vinegar. Enjoy!

29. Baked Sweet Potato Fritters: Preheat oven to 425°F. Place 2 sweet potatoes in a large bowl. Mash until smooth. Add 1/4 cup of diced onion, 1/4 cup of diced bell pepper, 1 teaspoon of garlic powder, and 1 egg. Mix until combined. Form into fritters and place on a lightly greased baking sheet. Bake for 20 minutes, or until fritters are golden brown. Enjoy!

30. Broiled Halibut with Asparagus: Preheat oven to broil. Place a piece of halibut in a baking dish. Top with a few sprigs of asparagus and 1 tablespoon of olive oil. Broil for 8 minutes, or until halibut is cooked through. Enjoy!

Chapter 6: Snack Recipes

1. Baked Apples: Preheat oven to 350°F. Core and slice 2 apples, and place them in a shallow baking dish. Sprinkle

with cinnamon, nutmeg, and a tablespoon of honey. Bake for 25-30 minutes, or until apples are tender. Serve warm.

2. Cucumber Salad: In a medium bowl, combine 1 cucumber (sliced), 1/2 cup of diced red onion, 2 tablespoons of olive oil, and 1 tablespoon of lemon juice. Toss to combine. Season with salt and pepper, to taste.

3. Oven Baked Zucchini Fries: Preheat oven to 425°F. Cut 1 zucchini into thin strips, and spread out on a baking sheet lined with parchment paper. Drizzle with 2 tablespoons of olive oil, and sprinkle with garlic powder, onion powder, and black pepper. Bake for 25-30 minutes, flipping halfway through. Serve warm.

4. Baked Sweet Potato Chips: Preheat oven to 425°F. Slice 1 sweet potato into thin slices. Place slices on a baking sheet lined with parchment paper, and drizzle with 2 tablespoons of olive oil. Sprinkle with garlic powder, onion powder, and salt, to taste. Bake for 25-30 minutes, flipping halfway through. Serve warm.

5. Avocado Toast: Toast 2 slices of whole grain bread. Mash 1/2 an avocado, and spread it on the toast. Sprinkle with a pinch of salt and pepper, to taste.

6. Hummus and Veggies: Slice up your favorite vegetables (carrots, celery, bell peppers, etc.) and dip them into a store-bought or homemade hummus.

7. Roasted Chickpeas: Preheat oven to 375°F. Drain and rinse 1 can of chickpeas, and place them on a baking sheet lined with parchment paper. Drizzle with 2 tablespoons of olive oil, and sprinkle with garlic powder, onion powder, and black pepper. Bake for 25-30 minutes, stirring halfway through. Let cool before serving.

8. Greek Yogurt Parfait: In a bowl or jar, layer 1/2 cup of Greek yogurt, 1/4 cup of berries, and 1/4 cup of granola. Repeat the layers one more time, and enjoy.

9. Egg Salad: In a medium bowl, mash 2 hard-boiled eggs. Add 2 tablespoons of plain Greek yogurt, 2 tablespoons of diced celery, and 1 tablespoon of diced red onion. Season with salt and pepper, to taste.

10. Fruit and Nut Bars: In a food processor, pulse together 1 cup of walnuts, 1 cup of almonds, 1/2 cup of dates, and 1/4 cup of coconut flakes until you get a crumbly consistency. Press the mixture into an 8×8-inch baking pan lined with

parchment paper. Refrigerate for at least 1 hour before slicing.

11. Baked Falafel: Preheat oven to 375°F. In a food processor, pulse 1 can of chickpeas, 1/2 cup of diced red onion, 2 cloves of garlic, 1 tablespoon of cumin, 1 tablespoon of coriander, 1/4 cup of parsley, and 1/4 cup of breadcrumbs until you get a crumbly mixture. Form the mixture into 1-inch balls and place them on a baking sheet lined with parchment paper. Bake for 20-25 minutes, or until golden brown.

12. Cottage Cheese and Berries: In a small bowl, combine 1/2 cup of cottage cheese with 1/4 cup of your favorite berries. Sprinkle with a pinch of cinnamon, and enjoy.

13. Spinach and Mushroom Quiche: Preheat oven to 375°F. Grease a 9-inch pie plate with 1 tablespoon of olive oil. In a medium bowl, mix together 1 cup of cooked spinach, 1/2 cup of diced mushrooms, 1/4 cup of diced red onion, 1/4 cup of shredded cheese, and 4 eggs. Pour the mixture into the prepared pie plate, and bake for 25-30 minutes, or until the center is set.

14. Roasted Carrots: Preheat oven to 375°F. Peel and cut 1 pound of carrots into 1-inch slices. Place them on a baking sheet lined with parchment paper. Drizzle with 2 tablespoons of olive oil, and sprinkle with garlic powder, onion powder, and black pepper. Bake for 25-30 minutes, flipping halfway through. Serve warm.

15. Green Smoothie: In a blender, combine 1 cup of spinach, 1 frozen banana, 1/2 cup of almond milk, and 1/2 cup of ice. Blend until smooth, and enjoy.

16. Egg Muffin Cups: Preheat oven to 375°F. Grease a 12-cup muffin tin with 1 tablespoon of olive oil. Crack 1 egg into each muffin cup, and top with a sprinkle of cheese and diced vegetables, if desired. Bake for 15-20 minutes, or until the eggs are set.

17. Baked Fish: Preheat oven to 375°F. Place 1 fillet of fish in a shallow baking dish, and season with salt and pepper, to taste. Drizzle with 1 tablespoon of olive oil, and bake for 25-30 minutes, or until the fish is cooked through.

18. Roasted Cauliflower: Preheat oven to 375°F. Cut 1 head of cauliflower into florets and spread out on a baking sheet lined with parchment paper. Drizzle with 2 tablespoons of

olive oil, and sprinkle with garlic powder, onion powder, and black pepper. Bake for 25-30 minutes, flipping halfway through. Serve warm.

19. Hummus and Veggie Wrap: Spread 2 tablespoons of hummus on a whole grain wrap. Top with your favorite vegetables, and roll up.

20. Greek Yogurt with Granola and Fruit: In a bowl, combine 1/2 cup of Greek yogurt with 2 tablespoons of granola and 1/4 cup of your favorite fruit. Enjoy.

21. Celery Sticks with Almond Butter: Cut 2 celery stalks into 3-inch pieces. Spread 1 tablespoon of almond butter on each piece, and enjoy.

22. Baked Oatmeal Cups: Preheat oven to 350°F. Grease a 12-cup muffin tin with 1 tablespoon of olive oil. In a medium bowl, whisk together 2 eggs, 1/2 cup of almond milk, 1/4 cup of honey, 1 teaspoon of vanilla extract, 1 teaspoon of cinnamon, and 1/4 teaspoon of salt. Add in 1 cup of rolled oats, and mix until combined. Divide the mixture into the prepared muffin tin, and bake for 25-30 minutes, or until the tops are golden. Let cool before serving.

23. Turkey Roll-Ups: Spread 1 tablespoon of cream cheese on a slice of deli turkey. Top with a few slices of cucumber, and roll up.

24. Asian Cucumber Salad: In a medium bowl, combine 1 cucumber (sliced), 2 tablespoons of rice vinegar, 1 tablespoon of soy sauce, 1 teaspoon of sesame oil, and 1 teaspoon of honey. Toss to combine.

25. Baked Sweet Potato Fries: Preheat oven to 425°F. Cut 1 sweet potato into thin strips, and spread out on a baking sheet lined with parchment paper. Drizzle with 2 tablespoons of olive oil, and sprinkle with garlic powder, onion powder, and black pepper. Bake for 25-30 minutes, flipping halfway through. Serve warm.

26. Apple Chips: Preheat oven to 375°F. Core and slice 1 apple, and spread out on a baking sheet lined with parchment paper. Sprinkle with cinnamon, nutmeg, and a pinch of salt. Bake for 25-30 minutes, flipping halfway through. Let cool before serving.

27. Tuna Salad: In a medium bowl, combine 1 can of tuna, 1/4 cup of diced celery, 2 tablespoons of plain Greek yogurt,

and 1 tablespoon of diced red onion. Season with salt and pepper, to taste.

28. Turkey Lettuce Wraps: Spread 2 tablespoons of hummus on a leaf of lettuce. Top with a few slices of deli turkey, and roll up.

29. Roasted Eggplant: Preheat oven to 375°F. Slice 1 eggplant into 1-inch slices and spread out on a baking sheet lined with parchment paper. Drizzle with 2 tablespoons of olive oil, and sprinkle with garlic powder, onion powder, and black pepper. Bake for 25-30 minutes, flipping halfway through. Serve warm.

30. Fruit Salad: In a medium bowl, combine 1 cup of diced pineapple, 1/2 cup of diced mango, 1/2 cup of blueberries, and 1/4 cup of diced kiwi. Drizzle with 1 tablespoon of honey, and toss to combine.

# Smoothie Recipe

1. Kale and Apple Smoothie: Blend 1 cup of kale, 1/2 cup of plain Greek yogurt, 1/2 cup of apple juice, and 1/2 cup of diced apple.

2. Carrot and Orange Smoothie: Blend 1 cup of carrot juice, 1/2 cup of orange juice, 1/2 cup of banana, and 1/4 cup of plain Greek yogurt.

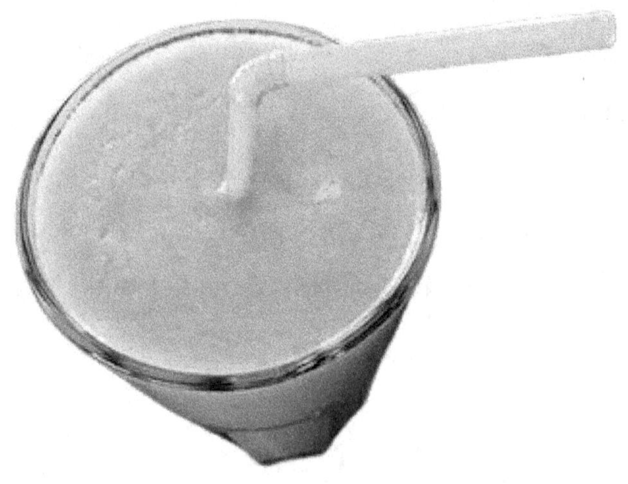

3. Banana and Almond Milk Smoothie: Blend 1 banana, 1/2 cup of almond milk, 1/4 cup of oats, and 1/4 cup of plain Greek yogurt.

4. Pumpkin and Pear Smoothie: Blend 1/2 cup of pumpkin puree, 1/2 cup of pear juice, 1/4 cup of plain Greek yogurt, and 1/4 cup of diced pear.

5. Cranberry and Coconut Smoothie: Blend 1/2 cup of cranberry juice, 1/2 cup of coconut milk, 1/4 cup of plain Greek yogurt, and 1/4 cup of shredded coconut.

6. Mango and Ginger Smoothie: Blend 1 cup of mango, 1/2 cup of orange juice, 1 teaspoon of grated ginger, and 1/4 cup of plain Greek yogurt.

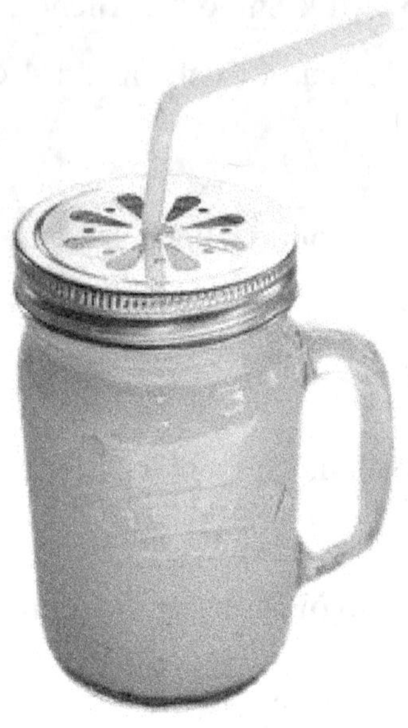

7. Peach and Chia Seed Smoothie: Blend 1 cup of peaches, 1/2 cup of almond milk, 1 tablespoon of chia seeds, and 1/4 cup of plain Greek yogurt.

8. Avocado and Spinach Smoothie: Blend 1/2 cup of avocado, 1/2 cup of almond milk, 1 cup of spinach, and 1/4 cup of plain Greek yogurt.

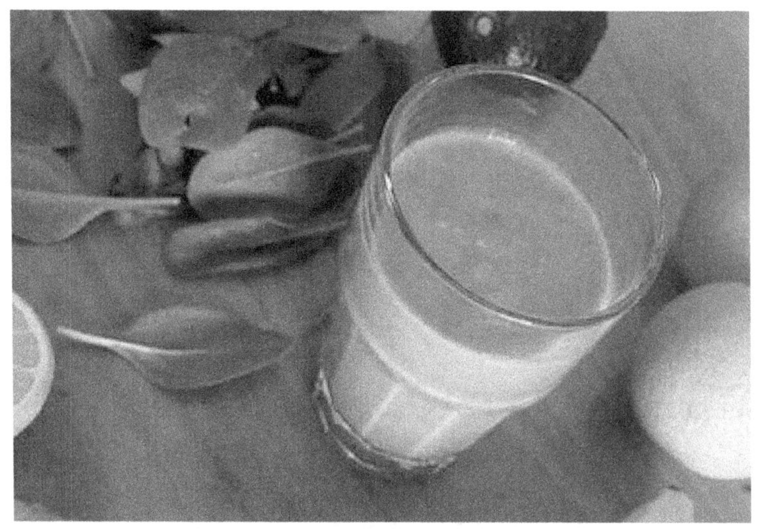

9. Apple and Cucumber Smoothie: Blend 1/2 cup of apple juice, 1/2 cup of cucumber juice, 1/4 cup of plain Greek yogurt, and 1/4 cup of diced apple.

10. Blueberry and Flaxseed Smoothie: Blend 1 cup of blueberries, 1/2 cup of almond milk, 1 tablespoon of flaxseed, and 1/4 cup of plain Greek yogurt.

11. Strawberry and Oat Smoothie: Blend 1 cup of strawberries, 1/2 cup of almond milk, 1/4 cup of oats, and 1/4 cup of plain Greek yogurt.

12. Banana and Cacao Smoothie: Blend 1 banana, 1/2 cup of almond milk, 1 tablespoon of cacao powder, and 1/4 cup of plain Greek yogurt.

13. Watermelon and Coconut Smoothie: Blend 1 cup of watermelon, 1/2 cup of coconut milk, 1/4 cup of plain Greek yogurt, and 1/4 cup of shredded coconut.

14. Pineapple and Flaxseed Smoothie: Blend 1 cup of pineapple, 1/2 cup of almond milk, 1 tablespoon of flaxseed, and 1/4 cup of plain Greek yogurt.

15. Raspberry and Almond Butter Smoothie: Blend 1 cup of raspberries, 1/2 cup of almond milk, 1 tablespoon of almond butter, and 1/4 cup of plain Greek yogurt.

16. Melon and Chia Seed Smoothie: Blend 1/2 cup of cantaloupe, 1/2 cup of almond milk, 1 tablespoon of chia seeds, and 1/4 cup of plain Greek yogurt.

17. Honeydew and Coconut Smoothie: Blend 1/2 cup of honeydew, 1/2 cup of coconut milk, 1/4 cup of plain Greek yogurt, and 1/4 cup of shredded coconut.

18. Peach and Oat Smoothie: Blend 1 cup of peaches, 1/2 cup of almond milk, 1/4 cup of oats, and 1/4 cup of plain Greek yogurt.

19. Banana and Coconut Smoothie: Blend 1 banana, 1/2 cup of coconut milk, 1 tablespoon of chia seeds, and 1/4 cup of plain Greek yogurt.

20. Kale and Pear Smoothie: Blend 1 cup of kale, 1/2 cup of pear juice, 1/4 cup of plain Greek yogurt, and 1/4 cup of diced pear.

21. Carrot and Apple Smoothie: Blend 1 cup of carrot juice, 1/2 cup of apple juice, 1/2 cup of banana, and 1/4 cup of plain Greek yogurt.

22. Mango and Oat Smoothie: Blend 1 cup of mango, 1/2 cup of almond milk, 1/4 cup of oats, and 1/4 cup of plain Greek yogurt.

23. Avocado and Orange Smoothie: Blend 1/2 cup of avocado, 1/2 cup of orange juice, 1/4 cup of plain Greek yogurt, and 1/4 cup of diced apple.

24. Blueberry and Coconut Smoothie: Blend 1 cup of blueberries, 1/2 cup of coconut milk, 1/4 cup of plain Greek yogurt, and 1/4 cup of shredded coconut.

25. Pumpkin and Banana Smoothie: Blend 1/2 cup of pumpkin puree, 1/2 cup of almond milk, 1/2 banana, and 1/4 cup of plain Greek yogurt.

26. Cranberry and Oat Smoothie: Blend 1/2 cup of cranberry juice, 1/2 cup of almond milk, 1/4 cup of oats, and 1/4 cup of plain Greek yogurt.

27. Watermelon and Flaxseed Smoothie: Blend 1 cup of watermelon, 1/2 cup of almond milk, 1 tablespoon of flaxseed, and 1/4 cup of plain Greek yogurt.

28. Honeydew and Apple Smoothie: Blend 1/2 cup of honeydew, 1/2 cup of apple juice, 1/4 cup of plain Greek yogurt, and 1/4 cup of diced apple.

29. Strawberry and Almond Butter Smoothie: Blend 1 cup of strawberries, 1/2 cup of almond milk, 1 tablespoon of almond butter, and 1/4 cup of plain Greek yogurt.

30. Melon and Chia Seed Smoothie: Blend 1/2 cup of cantaloupe, 1/2 cup of almond milk, 1 tablespoon of chia seeds, and 1/4 cup of plain Greek yogurt.

## FOODS TO AVOID

### 1. Fried or fatty foods

Fried or fatty foods are bad for the gastric system because they can increase the risk of developing **Gastroesophageal Reflux Disease** (GERD). GERD is a condition where the contents of the stomach reflux back up into the esophagus, causing heartburn and other symptoms. Fatty foods can contribute to this by relaxing the **Lower Esophageal Sphincter** (LES), which is the muscle that separates the stomach from the esophagus. When the LES is relaxed, it allows stomach acid and contents to reflux back up into the esophagus, causing GERD.

### 2. Spicy foods

Spicy foods can be bad for the gastric system because they can irritate the stomach lining and cause indigestion. They can also trigger the release of stomach acid, which can lead to heartburn.

In addition, spicy foods can speed up the movement of food through the digestive system, which can cause diarrhea. And finally, spicy foods can stimulate the release of the stress hormone cortisol, which can have a negative impact on the digestive system.

## 3. Alcohol

Alcohol is bad for the gastric system because it can irritate the lining of the stomach, which can lead to gastritis. Alcohol can also increase the production of stomach acid, which can further irritate the stomach lining and lead to ulcers.

## 4. Carbonated beverages

Carbonated beverages are bad for the gastric system because they can cause bloating, gas, and stomach pain. Carbonated beverages can also irritate the stomach lining and lead to indigestion.

Carbonated beverages should be avoided if you have a sensitive stomach or if you are prone to indigestion. If you must drink a carbonated beverage, drink it with a meal to help reduce the chances of stomach upset.

## 6. Citrus fruits

Citrus fruits are acidic in nature and can irritate the gastric system. This can lead to problems like heartburn, indigestion, and ulcers.

Citrus fruits are also high in sugar content. This can cause an increase in acid production in the stomach, which can further aggravate the gastric system.

Thus, it is best to avoid citrus fruits if you have a sensitive stomach or suffer from any gastric problems.

## 7. Beans and legumes

Beans and legumes can be difficult to digest due to their high fiber content. Additionally, they contain compounds called oligosaccharides which can cause gas and bloating. For people with sensitive stomachs, beans and legumes can be a trigger for digestive issues.

There are a few ways to make beans and legumes more digestible. Soaking them overnight can help to break down

**101 |THE GASTRIC DIET COOKBOOK**

some of the complex carbohydrates. You can also cook them with digestive-friendly herbs and spices like ginger, garlic, and turmeric. If you still find that beans and legumes cause digestive discomfort, it may be best to avoid them altogether

## 8. Sugary foods and beverages

Sugary foods and beverages can cause a number of problems for the gastric system. They can increase the risk of tooth decay, as well as contribute to obesity and other chronic health conditions. Additionally, they can cause heartburn and other discomfort.

There are a number of reasons why sugary foods and beverages are bad for the gastric system. First, they can increase the risk of tooth decay. When sugar is consumed, it can adhere to the teeth and form plaque. Over time, this plaque can lead to tooth decay.

Second, sugary foods and beverages can contribute to obesity. When people consume too many calories from sugar, they can gain weight. This extra weight can put strain on the entire body, including the gastric system.

Third, sugary foods and beverages can cause heartburn. When the stomach produces too much acid, it can lead to heartburn. This can be uncomfortable and can even lead to other health problems.

Fourth, sugary foods and beverages can cause other gastrointestinal problems. They can contribute to constipation and diarrhea. Additionally, they can upset the balance of good and bad bacteria in the gut, which can lead to other health problems.

Overall, sugary foods and beverages can cause a number of problems for the gastric system. They are best avoided, or consumed in moderation.

# CHAPTER 5

## Conclusion

Going on a gastric diet is important because it can help you maintain a healthy weight, reduce your risk of developing chronic health conditions, and improve your overall quality of life. Eating a balanced gastric diet can also reduce your risk of developing certain types of cancer, such as colon and stomach cancer. Following a gastric diet can help you to achieve and maintain a healthy weight, which can help you look and feel your best.

Overall, a gastric diet is essential to maintaining a healthy lifestyle. Not only can it help you maintain a healthy weight, but it can also reduce your risk of developing certain chronic health conditions. Eating a balanced gastric diet can also reduce your risk of developing certain types of cancer. Furthermore, following a gastric diet can help you to achieve and maintain a healthy weight, which can improve your overall quality of life.